Other titles by **SHARNY ❤ JULIUS**

FIT, HEALTHY HAPPY MUM

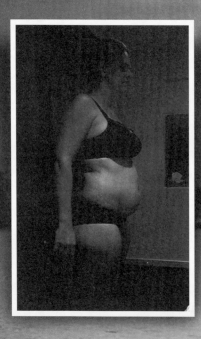

HOW MY QUEST FOR
PERFECT BREASTMILK
HELPED ME LOSE
24 KILOS IN ONLY
EIGHT WEEKS AFTER
THE BIRTH OF MY
FOURTH CHILD.

SHARNY ⊗ JULIUS

www.sharnyandjulius.com

FITmum by SHARNY ✂ JULIUS

How my quest for perfect breatmilk helped me lose 24 kilos in only 8 weeks after the birth of my fourth child

www.sharnyandjulius.com
email:sharnyandjulius@sharnyandjulius.com

Copyright © the Kieser Publishing Trust
First published by Kieser Publishing Trust in June 2013

Front Cover Photography: Captured by Bec

Front Cover Photography: sharnyandjulius

Typesetting and Design: sharnyandjulius

ISBN: 978-0-9871428-5-6

Before We Begin

In this book, I use the word husband, because that is what I have, so when I say husband, please read it as whatever you have, be it partner, wife, hubby, friend, lover, whatever. When you read marriage, read it as whatever relationship you have with your partner.

Also, when I refer to your child, I refer to it as a 'him', because once again I am relating to my first hand experience, my last child was a boy. Please read it as 'her' if you have a girl!

SHARNY 𝕾 JULIUS

Focus on the pursuit of excellence leading to mastery. This should be the purpose of your life, or you could cop out and just choose to be a passenger.

Start on the journey for health mastery and the seeds of excellence will invariably creep into the rest of your life, showing up in unexpected, but remarkable ways.

SHARNY ❤ JULIUS

Contents

Fuck it

I can't think of where it started. Running through scenarios can't seem to bring up the definitive point in time that I decided to say 'fuck it'. Maybe it was running through my head all along. Maybe it was when I met Julius and his alienation of victimisation has entrenched itself into my persona.

Kind of like a leech, but a good one. He'll say he's a leech, he'll say he's turned me into the modern day version of the scarlet letter. But maybe not. Maybe it was me. I'm a mother after all, I'm a woman and by virtue that means I do what I please. When I please.

And then I fell pregnant. All the power in me went out. Like a light I was snuffed. "You can't do this, you can't do that"… Like waves on a rising tide, everyone had advice for me. From family, friends and professionals to total strangers.

All conflicting, all compelling, mostly idle chatter, but when you add up the idle chatter, when you add up the waves upon waves upon waves, you can carve the biggest, most powerful cliff face to dust.

Well, to me, that's what happened. A strong, powerful woman who believed she had everything under a semblance of control. To a weak, meek, victim, cowering in the corner questioning everything I did, then second guessing it. Then feeling guilty. Then feeling guilty about being guilty, and so on and so on until I just gave up.

It may have been just me. It certainly felt like it was just me.

The solution I came up with was to take the passenger seat.

In everything.

You know how you feel like you are driving your life? All things you do are proactive, and the results and reactions happen to other people? Well, falling pregnant (and even more so, having a baby) drove me, wave by wave into the passenger seat. What was once a proactive, productive life became a reactive, desolate life of "what next".

I would wake in the morning at some ungodly hour, stinking. The thought of showering had not even registered, because that would be proactive. Right then, there is a screaming baby wanting a feed. Easy, I'd just do that. While sitting there in the creaky chair, I would just blank out, like a computer waiting for a virus. "What next".

"What clothes should I wear today?" I'd ask Julius.

"Whatever you want to wear" was his pragmatic response, followed by a querisome look.

If I hadn't been in such an open, reactive state, I would have thought, "he doesn't get it, he doesn't know how hard it is to make the right decision." But I didn't even think that. Like a robot, I'd just repeat myself "what clothes should I wear today," and then in a different way until he gave me an answer. Another decision I didn't have to make for myself. Another decision I didn't have to get wrong.

Before long, I'd moved myself from the passenger seat to the back seat, to the boot.

Fear. It was all fear. New mum indecision. Think about vaccination for a minute. If you don't vaccinate, your child will risk dying. If you do, however, you risk your child dying overnight from the vaccine. Looking into this debate each way is a scary thing to do. Both ways have horrific stories.

We nearly lost Alexis the night after her 2-month vaccination. Sitting in the bottom of a freezing shower trying to cool down my overheating, screaming baby was scary. When she went quiet, looked into the distance and started to convulse? Even remembering that makes my heart stop.

Seeing the desperate looks on the paramedics faces as they wrapped her in ice from the freezer... Back into the reactive state. The boot. It's safe there. You can't make a wrong decision in there; you simply don't make any decisions.

And then one day, I got through that vapid, exhaustive, waif like state and realised that everyone else had moved on except me. My babies were older and hardier. My husband was still there, but didn't really look at me any more. He's too busy making all the decisions. All the decisions that I was afraid to make.

One look in the mirror and I saw the result of this vegetative state. I looked like a hippo. A fat hippo. A fat, hairy, regrowth, pale hippo. And *old*.

Oh no. I remember thinking. That beautiful, powerful, decisive woman you were has grown old and tired. And fat. Who is this tired, angry looking woman staring back at me? It looks like me, if I was a witch.

Maybe this is where I should have said, "fuck it". But I didn't because 2 lines on the pregnancy test meant that I was thrown straight back into the hurricane.

Somewhere then and now, I remember looking in the mirror and seeing the old lady again. She had been feeding well.

Slip, like time moving sideways I went back into my safe little cube in time to see the world go by like when you let your attention go as you look out the side of a car.

And then somewhere I decided to say, "fuck it". Normally I don't swear, but I cannot think of a more potent, poignant way to say it. "Fuck it".

Say it now (it's especially delicious if you normally don't swear).

"Fuck it".

And with those two words my life changed. And so should yours…

A Tropical Island

Right now is the time you will want to put the book down and move back to your cube. But just for a moment, please don't.

I want you to have a chance to see what I have now. Hang in there with me for a moment, I promise that I will not waste your time. I know what it's like being a new mum. *I know.*

If you feel like a boat, lost at sea in a horrendous storm, a storm that nobody else can see or appreciate, then I promise you that the stories I am about to share with you will be like a tropical island. Complete with hours of uninterrupted massage and pampering.

If you really don't have the time, call your mother, your best friend or whoever you can. Tell them this:

"I need out for the morning. I'm not me anymore and I just need to reconnect with me so that I can get out of this vegetative state. Mum, please, could you look after the kids for the morning. I need you right now."

Once you've convinced her to do it, get in your car and drive out to get a haircut. Get a dramatic change. Get your colour done. Do something crazy!

Then settle in to the rest of this book.

What's in the book

In this book, I will share with you my story of how I started as a fat, middle aged mother, with no motivation, no time, no sex drive and no self respect, and finished with a life that I couldn't even conjure up in a fantasy, only 8 weeks after the birth of my 4th child.

I'll share with you

- How I have more time now, with 4 kids than I ever did before having any kids.

- How I lost over 24 kilograms in the 8 weeks after the birth of my 4th baby

- Why I can actually run properly now

- How I get more done in 2 hours than I used to do in a whole week

- How I used sex to get a more powerful pelvic floor

- Why having a baby can make you more capable of multiple orgasms

- Why you should be flaunting your stretch marks, not hiding them

- How you can (and should) become the queen in your life, not the slave

A little about me

My name is Sharny Kieser and I live in a little seaside holiday town on the Sunshine Coast in Australia. Nowadays, my husband and I make a living out of writing fitness books and spend most of my time flying around the country to talk about our 'controversial' opinions on various fitness topics.

As I write this book, I have 4 kids and one to go.

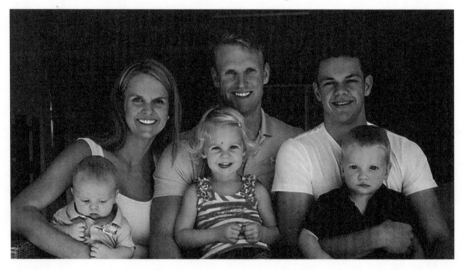

Josh is 16

Alexis is 2 ½

Danté is 1 ½

Emmett is 15 weeks old

I had my first child at the age of 16. Most people would have written me off as trash (even I did) because of being a teen mum. Josh, my amazing, beautiful son is 16 now, and has been the strength in my life since he was born.

A few years later (a little older but not much wiser) we were waiting for the right time to grow the family, when it happened. I fell pregnant with Alexis. We'd planned to have 4 more kids straight after one another, so we kind of 'fell into it'.

When I fell pregnant with Alexis, I swore I wouldn't put on any weight. I had a fitness gym at the time and we were writing our first book *Never Diet Again*.

That's when I became fat. Then fatter, then fatter. It's not nice becoming fat, especially being a fitness *expert*. I use the word *expert* loosely, because I certainly didn't feel like one, I had no qualifications to be one and the most important qualification (my body) was slowly getting covered in a thick layer of fat.

I was eating myself to death. I would love to blame someone, at the time I blamed everyone else, but the truth is that it was all me. We have helped thousands of people escape the diet trap forever, and they never get there until they make the distinction that getting fat was all their fault, so losing the fat is all their responsibility.

At the time I was certainly not living my word. Practicing what I preach. I had heard the saying "you're eating for two" and preferred that.

Before falling pregnant with Alexis, I was around 60kg with abs and a big butt. 2 days after I had birthed Emmett (15 weeks ago) I stood on the scales to find I was 84kilos (the same weight as when I fell pregnant with him, so couldn't even blame baby weight!)

8 weeks later, I weighed 60kilos and now I weight 58 kilos, I'm fitter than I have been in a long time, I'm nearly as strong as I ever have been, I have lost my big bum (surprise!) and the best part is that I am the happiest I have ever been.

I used to think of having kids as a kind of inevitable 'giving up' on my life. Of sacrificing myself for my kids. I want to share with you how that is totally the opposite to what having kids is all about and why having kids should give you energy, not take it away…

A Patch of Heather

Why?

What a great question. Why is it that we as mums sacrifice our own identities, our own lives for our families?

To find out why, I first needed to know what benefit we have from being this way. The common misconception is that being a mum, you have to give up your life for your kids, right?

You have to give up.

You have to give up… your *life*.

I had the good fortune of talking in depth to a war veteran the other day. He told me of one battle that changed his life. Him and his battalion had been ambushed on the road to a small town, early in the morning. As his friends and comrades were gunned down in front of him and around him, he threw himself onto the ground.

He told me that to mentally survive the carnage of a battle, he had been told to focus on the small things that mattered. It was tempting to stare at the gruesome scenes around him, captivated by the horror of it all, let go and just succumb to the madness.

Through a small stroke of good fortune, he had fallen into a patch of heather. As his eyes faded through the grotesque scenes around him and ahead of him, he shortened his focus to the flowers. As he lay there, he became mesmerised by the simple beauty of the tiny purple flowers, standing tall in defiance and complete contrast to the environment around them.

In that moment, he was literally overcome with this feeling that all would be well. Instead of giving up his life, he released his tensions and relaxed, he felt at peace and at ease. His words were "I am going to die here, in hell, so with every last breath I choose to only see the beauty of it."

And with that *decision*, things changed for him.

Outside his immediate view were more flowers, bright and defiant and beautiful. Beyond the whistling and drum drum of war, he could hear his heart beating. A beautiful sound among all the death.

With every breath he grew happier and happier until he began to hum. And then sing. In the middle of a war scene he sang, louder and louder. After a few verses, he heard others joining him. Within a few minutes, the song had infected the whole battlefield, guns stopped firing as even the enemy paused to listen to this joyful madness. Looking up he saw a V of geese flying overhead in a bright blue sky, unaware or not caring about what was happening below.

In those moments, he felt happier than he had in his entire life.

And that is how it was for me. And it can be for you too.

It is so easy to focus on the chaos, the lack of sleep, the constant crying, and the continuous barrage of horror stories. It's expected of you.

But it's just as easy to overlook it like the war veteran, and see only the beauty. Because before you know it, the intensity of the situation fades and then goes away. Every disaster goes away. Every war ends.

All that is left are the scars.

And for a mum, they can be emotional, like PND. Or they can be physical, like getting fat.

But unlike war, scars can be avoided. It's as simple as a *choice*.

And that is what this book is about. I'm no supermum, I'm no hero, I just decided that because it was how it was always done, didn't mean I had to accept it.

And I didn't. And neither should you.

This book is not a 'how to' or a way for me to preach to you. It's a way for me to share my story with you, like a sister. I won't hold anything back, I have no agenda other than to share the possibilities I have been fortunate to experience.

By doing so, I hope that you will be inspired to see that you are so much more than "just a mother". You can have kids and a career. You can have kids and a body to die for. You can have kids and stay sane. You can have no sleep and still perform. You can have a family, and keep your identity.

In fact, if you have kids, if you have a family or are about to – you *have to* keep your identity. You absolutely, positively *must* keep your identity.

Which brings us to the "why". And here is a very powerful why.

The Slave and the Queen

If you believe the idea that being a mum means that you put everyone ahead of you, then ask yourself this question.

If I put everybody ahead of me, what am I?

Answer: a slave.

Now try this:

Who puts themselves before everyone else?

Answer: a queen

Let's continue this line of questioning:

If you don't look after yourself, will you be able to look after your kids?

Here's the kicker. A question that blew my mind and changed my life.

Who has more influence? A slave or a queen?

If you treat yourself like a slave, you will be treated like a slave. If you treat yourself with importance, like a queen, you will be respected.

Who do your kids want as a parent… a *slave*, or a *queen*?

Would you want your mother to have been… a *slave*, or a *queen*?

Being a queen doesn't mean that everyone sacrifices for you. It means that you put your wellbeing first, because you *know* that to do so will make you a better queen, a better provider, a better wife, a better person... a better mother.

And by god it does.

A Note from My Husband

I want to see more stretch marks.

I love stretch marks. I think that nothing symbolises womanhood more than a tummy criss-crossed with those pale crescents of beauty.

I've never really understood the attraction to young, flawless models. As a boy, I always preferred the company of people older than me; there is something so appealing about life experience. I can appreciate natural gifted perfection, but wow, the intrigue and depth of character of age and experience gets my soul singing.

Maybe that is why I love athletes so much. If I were to pinpoint it, my attraction to someone is directly proportional to how hard they have had to work, how much they have had to sacrifice.

And when I say sexy or attractive, I don't mean that I want to jump on you and dry hump your leg. Because there is an electricity that a man or woman of life experience emits. An edginess to their voice, a deep sense of self that emanates from them. An attractiveness that cannot be faked by immaturity.

Think about Seal for example. Facial scars like his cannot be hidden. The personal torment he has had to go through to just show his face at a young age, when they began, has created a strength of character that is magnetic. Millions of women around the world find him irresistible. Sexy.

Real beauty in my opinion is a direct result of hard work, of sacrifice. Be it emotional or physical. Being born perfect is an amazing gift, but hard work leaves signs. Scars. None sexier than stretch marks.

Sharn has had 4 kids so far (one more to go), and each time, in the aftermath of the birth, I feel like she has been reborn. Not physically, but her soul has gone on a journey alone – to a place where great experience is earned. She has this deep monk like calmness and contentedness that I find irresistible. Intriguing… sexy.

I for one am jealous that she (and you) can have the profound experience of something so intense and satisfying as birthing a child. Your child. I'm sure if you ask your husband, he'll choke back tears at the thought of how tough you are to have done that with such grace.

Maybe that's why men go to war. No act by a man will come close to matching the courage, strength and toughness carrying and birthing a child does, so we battle. But battle destroys lives. You sacrifice to create life.

Wow.

Apart from a beautiful baby that hopefully looks more like her than me, Sharny has earned a few stripes. When the belly has gone down and the shape has returned, which she's going to tell you how to do, she's left with her mummy badges.

And I *love* them. I wish she'd wear midriff shirts all the time. I'm so proud of her. No bikie patch, no war wound or tattoo will ever come close to the perfect symbol of strength that a mummy badge has.

A little bit of a tan and they change colour from purple to a pale brown. And it's not just her. If I catch a small glimpse of another mums mummy badges as she bends over to pick up her baby I can't help but look, take a moment and think about how powerful she is.

I have a scar on my rib cage. Not very big, but I show it off every chance I get. I tell people I got stabbed there trying to save a baby from a great white. I actually had a mole removed. 3 stitches. That's right. All my man friends show off their scars with pride.

All our scars are pathetic compared to birth scars. But you women feel like you should be ashamed of them? You should hide them?

I hope for your sake that as the intensity of birthing a child wears down to normality, you can have some stretch marks. Mummy badges. I hope for the sake of women around the world, and especially men who appreciate hard work as sexy, you show those bad boys off like your new cleavage.

Mummy badges. HOT!

Julius

Before The Baby Is Born

Have a Routine

One thing I cannot stress enough is that you're going to need a routine. Any routine, but a routine will make your life so much easier. I can't count the number of times that I have been on the verge of a breakdown only to revert back to thinking about the routine. *How many minutes to sleep time* is a calming thought when the stress of the day gets to a peak.

I for one cannot imagine how women cope without that thought, reactive parenting. Waiting until the baby decides it wants to sleep.

There are a couple of fantastic books to read if you want a routine that works; *Save our Sleep*, by Tizzie Hall, and *The Contented Little Baby* Book by Gina Ford.

They're both great resources to start with, but I found (and talking to a lot of friends) that while you may start with their routine as gospel, you quickly adapt it to suit your own style. The key though, is to *have a routine*.

Set some rules

Before we had all our kids, a friend of ours told us about their 8 week 'lockdown'. 8 weeks of no visitors.

We thought that it was selfish when we first heard about it, but after the first 2 days of endless visitors wanting to cuddle the baby - resulting in a very restless, distressed baby – we instigated the lock down.

I strongly recommend you do it. The hardest part is telling all those well-meaning people that they can't visit for a few weeks; but every one of them will understand. Better yet, get your husband to tell them.

We never ended up doing the full 8 weeks for any of our kids, and we did have some visitors; but having a blanket rule like this will make the visitors that you *do* have really appreciative of the fact that you 'bent the rules' for them. And they will, more importantly, not pester you for cuddles.

On a similar note, perfumes are an absolute no-no for visitors. Smell is the strongest and most important senses for your little baby. To be overwhelmed by *Chanel no 5* quite often means he will struggle to find your nipple later on, and subsequently get very stressed out.

We have one friend who refused to talk to us because Julius told her she couldn't come in. She called me recently after having her first baby to thank me for the great idea and to apologise for being so selfish at the time.

Week One

Let's get into week 1, what to expect and what to do from when you're left all on your own, with *a baby* to care for.

It's so weird the first few minutes. It always seems so surreal, like I'm holding someone else's baby, feeling like I'm not mature enough to care for something so beautiful and precious!

Before your baby is born, you are the centre of attention.

Everybody wants to wish you well, spend some time with you, share their war stories, check on you. Once the baby is born, you're dropped. As fast as the umbilical chord gets cut, the attention is diverted.

For some people that is exciting. For a new mum it can be the most eerie, surreal feeling. It certainly was for me. Leading into birth, I was surrounded by help, lured into this feeling of security. It was easy for me to believe that the obstetrician, and the midwives would be there afterwards.

Having them around so much during the birth and for the last 9 months, somehow got me subconsciously convinced that they would be there for the rest of my life. All of a sudden, the curtain is pulled back, the room cleared and you're left alone. Where before, the room was filled with chatter and movement, now all you hear is the sound of your breathing.

And your baby.

Your baby.

That's right. It's yours.

For me, this is the moment that the gravity and responsibility of it all hits me. Every single birth has been the same. It's the same feeling you get when you graduate school. Pregnancy is over. You're a mum now. This little bundle of grunts is wholly your responsibility for at least the next 20 years. And you've got NO support.

This baby is yours. All yours. "All bought and paid for" as Julius would say. The excitement and lead up is over, just like the day after your wedding. Maybe this is how PND starts. You realise how important it is that you don't mess up this child.

At least that's what runs through my head when the room finally goes quiet and all the people you have spent hours with, sharing intimate details of your anatomy just disappear out of your life.

Don't let it stress you out!

Take this as a perfect opportunity to reflect on your life. On how you have grown up, how you have just gone through the most intense experience of your entire life. You're unmistakably a woman now. Never again can someone treat you like a girl.

Think on that for a moment. You're not a girl anymore. You're a mother. And being a mother means you have power.

Side note: *I have some friends who never got over this feeling, they buckled under the feeling that their lives were never going to be the same again, their 'perfect life' was over. Don't worry, before you know it, your baby will fit into your life.*

Refuse to let PND into your life. Understand that every mother goes through an adjustment period. And if you think you won't, put it into perspective. A friend of mine had to turn the life support off on her baby when he was only 8 days old.

You're fine, your baby is fine. Everything will be fine!

So, in the interest of giving you some support (virtually), here are a few things to calm your nerves that nobody tells you about.

Sleeping, what's that?

You're not going to sleep. The hormones in your body won't allow it. Don't worry about missing sleep; you're going to be absolutely amazed at how little sleep you need.

Due to the magic of these hormones, your sleep requirements have gone from 8 hours a day down to about 2.

Pooing is going to be a challenge

Sitting on the toilet feeling like I had been kicked in the vagina by a horse, I would have killed to be able to poo.

I wish I had this much blockage *during* the birth - 9 out of 10 women poo during childbirth. Wish they'd told me that statistic before my 4th. I thought I was the only one with a butt-hole like a storm drain.

Part of the reason pooing is hard is because you have haemorrhoids. It sounds gross, but if you get a hand mirror out and watch yourself poo, you'll see what looks like rat testicles hanging out of your bum.

Once again, 9 out of 10 women have them. They go away (back inside) after a few weeks. You can get a cream for them and you'll need to push them back in after every poo…but not straight away. You'll have the pleasure of looking like a hermaphrodite for at least a week before they are able to be touched.

Julius doesn't find *them* sexy. He does think they're pretty funny though, especially when I'm wincing in pain, and telling him through gritted teeth "if this is what being kicked in the balls feels like, I am sympathetic."

Probably not a good idea to ask your husband to help push your "rats nuts" back in for you. Julius says its like getting dogs into a bath. As one gets in, the other jumps out.

Probiotic certainly helped me here. Get a good quality probiotic, a good idea anyway, and you won't feel like you're passing steel wool. It also helps your little baby to become regular.

Uterine contractions

Period pain? Meh, that's nothing compared to uterine contractions. As your uterus comes back down to normal size, it burns like the fires of hell. Your saving grace here is that you have just given birth to a watermelon - what's a little hell fire to a new mum?

One thing I will point out is that breastfeeding at this time brought on my uterine contractions. For the first 3 kids I struggled with breastfeeding, part of the reason was that subconsciously I associated feeding with the pain.

For baby 4, I was ready for it, and interestingly it wasn't as bad as I remembered.

Get your structure checked

Because we live so close to the ocean, anything metal rusts if left outside; The little screws in kids toys being the worst. I have lost count of the number of times I've seen Julius with a kitchen knife prying open the side of one of these toys to replace the batteries.

It's a delicate operation that requires brute strength and apparently a lot of sweating and swearing as he opens the seam, then gets his fingers in and without breaking the plastic gets the old batteries out and the new ones in, before pulling his hands away. With a clack, the two halves of the toy snap back into place.

That's kind of like what birthing does to your pelvic region. The forces are immense, as the seams are pulled apart against straining fibres. As soon as the baby comes through, it all 'snaps back' into place.

But because of the intricacies and the softness of the connective tissue, when it snaps back, like the toy, it could snap back slightly crooked.

Slightly crooked now may be alright because everything is so soft and the pain is miniscule in comparison to your other pains. But when everything else dies down, and the tissues tighten up again, a nerve that is slightly pinched can turn into agony as the bones close back onto each other like a vice.

So, while you're soft and malleable, have a chiropractor or osteopath look you over. Because of the softness of the tissues, it is a perfect time to move your pelvic joints around to realign you.

I have heard of many women who've been able to use the opportunity to fix other joint issues while the body is in "repair mode".

Eating for wellness (and good quality milk)

Through our time in the fitness industry, we've seen some amazing physical transformations. None more impressive than from Cancer sufferers.

You see, a Cancer sufferer does not eat to lose body weight, or for a better body image; they eat to survive. They eat for wellness.

We nearly lost Alexis, our daughter the night after her 2-month vaccination. As a result, we decided to stop vaccinating all together, something we didn't even know was possible.

We did our research and decided that the risks of death from vaccination were higher than the risk of death from the diseases we were vaccinating against.

Vaccination is a touchy subject. You're damned if you don't and you're damned if you do. Whatever you do choose, please have a compelling, self researched reason. Don't just follow the herd (and that's not a dig at vaccination, there are a growing number of self righteous people who don't vaccinate for the sake of anarchism - giving a bad name to people who have their own reasons not to vaccinate.)

While this book could spark a massive debate on vaccination, it's not the purpose, or the point.

So what is the point in bringing it up in the first place?

Well, because we decided not to vaccinate, it was imperative that we ensure our kids internal and external environment was not conducive to disease. Which is why we turned our attention, naturally, to wellness eating. The type of eating people do when they are dying, and the medical industry has run out of answers for them.

If a cancer sufferer, who has been told to say their goodbyes, can reverse their disease purely through eating for wellness, surely we can extrapolate those nutrition guidelines to little babies and breastfeeding mothers.

If they can turn back from death to health, what are the possibilities for someone who is healthy to start with?

So we did.

And do you know what cancer beaters eat? A chemical cocktail of supplements?

No.

Vegetables.

Lots of vegetables, as raw as they can.

And the best part of eating like this is that you can eat as much as you want. Portion control is a thing of the past.

Nutrition versus Calories

It's a pretty selfish woman who diets while breastfeeding. It's an even more stupid woman who says what I just said. The hormones in your body will NEVER let you restrict food to your baby.

It's getting fed, whether you like it or not. Cravings when breastfeeding are so much stronger than in pregnancy. But, and here is a big but, they are not random. Every breastfeeding woman I talk to feels hungry for the same thing. Nutrition.

When I had Alexis, I felt hungry *all* the time. My subconscious mind was telling me to get nutrition into my system, so that I could feed it to the baby. The problem was that my food had very little nutritional value.

When I say nutritional value, I mean essential vitamins and minerals, amino acids and other micronutrients that are carried in with the energy molecules of fat and carbs as well as proteins.

You see, a carbohydrate molecule and a fat molecule alone have no *nutritional* value to the body. They are only used for generating energy.

If you imagine your body as a house, carbs and fats are like firewood. They are used to generate *energy*. We need energy to survive. In the body, this firewood is called calories.

But a body, just like a house, needs more than calories to survive. Think about all the other things that have to come into your house every single day.

At the front door of the house is an alarm. The alarm has only one purpose - to tell the house owner that they need to bring something into the house. The alarm doesn't discriminate - it will go off if the firewood has run out, in exactly the same way as if a light bulb has blown or the toilet paper has run out.

In the body, this alarm is called hunger, and just like the alarm on our imaginary house, it doesn't discriminate. It just tells you that you are hungry, it doesn't tell you what you are hungry *for.*

So like the house, if you just keep bringing in firewood, when you've run out of toilet paper, the alarm is going to keep going off - no matter how much firewood you bring in.

If you just keep eating carbs, fats and proteins, you will continue to feel hungry, no matter how much you eat.

When you start to think about eating like this, your life will change forever.

Like the cancer sufferer, you will transition from malnourished but fat, to well nourished and thin. Your baby will become much easier to settle. I used to think Alexis and Danté were very fussy eaters, but now I know that their little alarms were yelling at them for nutrition, and all I was feeding them was calories.

Babies are so intuitive - when they need nutrition, but we feed them calories, they refuse to eat and get *fussy*. When we adults need nutrition, but are fed calories, we just keep eating and eating *the same thing*.

Insanity?

Flavour as an indicator of nutrition

Before, when I said that your alarm can't tell you what you need, but it can. You already have the capacity to tell what you need from your food. Your body just doesn't have a reference point.

Have you ever wondered why you like to eat different meals all the time? Most animals eat the exact same meal, sometimes 3 times a day, every single day their entire lives. Why do we struggle with having the same dinner two nights in a row?

While I used to think it was because of our advanced brain capacity for choice and control, the truth is a little more interesting than that.

Flavour is our indicator of nutrition. As humans, our environment has become far more than just eat, sleep and breed. As a result, our nutritional requirements are slightly (only slightly) more complex than our animal friends.

We want a variety of flavour, because our body need a variety of nutrition.

The problem we face, however, now that we know this, is that almost all the food we are eating is artificially flavoured and coloured. When we might need nutrient X, which is found only in green apples, we go looking for a green apple and in our minds eye we picture a delicious bright green apple.

But then the picture (almost instantly) gets replaced by a green jellybean. Much greener than a green apple, and far more 'green apple' tasting than a green apple. So we eat the jellybeans instead.

And what are jellybeans?

Firewood that has been painted to look like apples.

Cancer surviving wellness experts will tell you that it is the paint (the artificial flavours and colours) that are causing the most damage - because they are not food, they are chemicals.

So you have this double whammy. You needed nutrient X, but you end up with more calories, some poisonous additive, AND you never ended up getting your nutrient X - so you go back for more!

This is why people are always hungry, babies are fussy and mums are absolutely depleted.

As much as you love your baby, you need to understand that while he is breastfeeding, he is just like a parasite - he will get all his nutrition from you, at the expense of yours.

Eating food that is high calorie, low nutrition is going to wreck you internally, because your body will begin to shut down like a starvation victim, while at the same time you'll be getting fatter!

If you eat for wellness, you will not only have a baby that is content (because he is getting the nutrition he wants), but you will be satisfied - because you too, will have the nutrition your body craves.

And for some people, for the first time in their entire lives, they will not have that feeling of hunger that haunts their every waking hour.

Imagine that!

Set your reference point in the very first week

As I said before, your body already has the capacity to tell you what it needs or craves, you just need to provide it with that reference point.

Combine this with the fact that you are now solely responsible for providing your baby with all of its nutrition as well as all of yours. It's time to reset your body's flavour reference point.

This can be quite tricky and take a fair bit of time, because for a lot of us, we are very malnourished to begin with. But you'll begin to tell, because your cravings change dramatically, and the satiety, that feeling of contented fullness is almost instant; as opposed to that sick feeling of overeating calorie dense, nutrition poor food.

This process can take about 3 weeks to complete, but the results are near instantaneous; and if I was to be honest, it can become quite a passion, so talking about clean eating recipes with friends can become a massive focus of your life - for the rest of your life.

So how do you start?

It's simple. Sometime in the first week, get your husband to buy you a massive *variety* of vegetables. The sooner the better.

Remember that a great time for change is when everything is changing, so I'd say do it on day one, but if you don't get out of hospital for a few days, don't stress, just do it as soon as you can.

Get different types of vegetables, and also different colours of vegetables, then get him to pick out different shades of colour in the exact same vegetables.

Then get him to buy a variety of seeds and nuts.

When he brings it home, get him to lay it all out on the bench for you, take them out of their bags, wash them and display them in all their glory.

This is where the fun happens.

Look at them all. Your eyes will tell you what they want, based on the colour of the vegetable. Start making a salad, or a smoothie, or a juice (whatever you feel like making) with whatever coloured vegetables take your fancy.

You'll be absolutely amazed at what you come up with. If you are malnourished in a particular micronutrient, you'll binge eat on that colour vegetable until you no longer need that nutrient.

Combinations of different colours and flavours, when digested follow different chemical pathways in the body, so the options are literally endless. Have fun, play with it, make sure your husband joins in; the benefits will be felt almost instantaneously for both of you, and even more potently the longer you have been malnourished for!

Warning: Doing it this way will potentially waste a lot of food, but you cannot tell what you need until it is in front of you; so I won't tell if you don't.

Milk coming down

Eating a clean, vegetable rich diet will fix your nutrition, but you need to get the delivery right. Don't stress about this too much, because if your nutrition is right, your body will self regulate with hunger and thirst, but to start with, you will need to drink at least 4 litres of water a day.

I found it helped if I had sparkling water, and when your hubby buys you those veggies, get a bag of lemons and a bag of limes. Cut one of each up in the morning and leave them in the fridge. As you get your water through the day, just pop a sliver of lemon or lime into your glass.

Sparkling mineral water is very cheap too, only 80c for a 1.5 litre bottle from the supermarket. You just can't buy it cold, so have a few bottles in the fridge that you keep stocking up on.

Have your husband keep a keen eye on how many bottles you have left: If you are drinking 4 litre a day each, that's 5 and a half bottles a day. Make sure you have enough to last a few days - and keep on top of the cold ones.

It can be quite frustrating getting up for a late night feed only to find the fridge bare of any "sparkles"!

Week Two

Finishing week one can be like dying for some new mums. Hopefully, treating your body to good nutrition and lots of water, you will feel like week one was an empowering experience.

Your little cherub should be so different now; you'll be amazed at how fast they seem to have grown up already! You would have had and gotten rid of your first visitors and you would have stared at your precious little baby a million times, wondering at how you could love something so much.

The feeling of being a mum, really being a mum, should be settling in well now. And along with that comes the feeling of being trapped. Don't mistake it for being trapped by parenthood; the truth is you've not left your house for over a week - something you've probably never done before, and you are going stir crazy!

It's time to get outside

NOTE: depending on the type of birth you had, getting outside may take a little longer than one week, but generally with a natural, uncomplicated birth, day 7 is about the day you just feel like you need to get outside.

So get outside.

I'm sure you've chosen your pram, and your poor hubby (who is undoubtedly feeling a little useless right now) is quite excited about you taking the pram (that he built) out for a walk.

Tell him you'd love him to push it, but you're probably going to need it for support.

It's not going to be too comfortable, and you won't be going far, but getting outside, just walking to the end of the street with the pram will not only mean the world to you, but will set your baby up for being comfortable in the pram.

Notes on choosing a pram.

For the first few weeks, a capsule that clips out of the pram base and into the car seat, is heaven sent. We went through quite a few prams before we got the one we liked, and simply because we don't have to wake the baby up as we move it from car to pram and vice versa.

After about 3 months, as you become more athletic, we cannot go past a chariot (hit up their website: chariotcarriers.com.au) they are amazing for running with – Our chariot has bicycle tyres, suspension AND a sling that the baby is suspended in.

Julius and I have tested it, and because of this triple suspension thing, running along a dirt road produces less vibration on the baby than walking a normal pram on a footpath.

Seriously, I could fill a book with what I love about our chariot (we have the twin one, that also attaches to the back of a bike). Comparing the chariot to a pram is like comparing an iPhone to an old landline. Start saving now - you're going to wonder how you would have managed exercise before you got it.

PS... we used a bunch of ping-pong balls to test it out, not a baby!

The important thing to think about while walking is that firstly, you are getting outside and getting your baby used to travel in a pram. But just as importantly, you are retraining movement in your hip joints.

Remember that you are still malleable, your ligaments still soft, so how you walk now should be representative (as much as you can with a giant pad between your legs) of how you want to walk, and more importantly how you want to run later on.

All my life I've run like an awkward duck - for years I've tried to change my running style to be more 'natural' and more efficient. Having started the post birth rehabilitation process with my desired running style in mind, has made me (only 15 weeks on) able to run how I never could before having the baby.

The idea is that your body is like wet clay. You now have the chance to shape it in whatever way you want before the clay sets. Think of yourself as a pottery master, and design the body you want now, so that when the clay sets, it looks and performs exactly how you wanted it to.

While other mothers are feeling trapped by their post birth bodies, you're hopefully realising that having a child gives you a whole new world of opportunity. Your baby isn't the only one who has been born.

Try to make one feed a bottle feed

In a few weeks time, you're going to want to get out of the house and do some exercise sans baby, and hope that your husband will be able to care for the baby while you are away, should the baby wake up.

In four or five weeks time, it's going to be nearly impossible to ween your baby onto the bottle, unless you've set him up for it in the first few weeks.

You may never need to give him a bottle, but knowing that the option is there, especially should an emergency arise, will give you much comfort knowing that he will be able to still feed.

I would suggest starting this in week 2, while he is still not able to make the distinction between teat and nipple. So every day, I would express one feed (of about 60ml) that I would feed him through the bottle.

It is also a really good idea for this feed to be done by your husband, so that they get used to each other. It is really easy to be a 'baby hog' and it's hard letting go, but your baby needs to spend time with his daddy too (and it will give you a chance to do something else).

I expressed my feed at 9pm, and Julius would feed it to the baby at 2am when he started work. Alternately, your husband can feed it to him at say 10pm, when he goes to bed and you do the 2am feed if your husband is a late sleeper.

This really does help you as a mum to get quite a good sleep, and you will be so thankful for it in a few weeks time when you want to do something that requires you to be away for more than 15 minutes at a time!

Get in the shower

This has nothing to do with your body, but swimming teachers recommend that you get your baby in the shower as soon as possible - obviously you don't put their face under the faucet, but the sound and feel of the water will help them to transition to swimming a lot better later on.

I found that the shower is one of the best places to take an inconsolable baby. Time will tell if my theory works, but all of my kids now want to have a shower when they're stressed out.

A lot of my friends give their kids food when they are stressed out. I believe that this may be the earliest trigger of comfort eating - I'd certainly love it if when I was stressed out, I craved a swim or shower instead of chocolate!

Eating in week 2

By week 2, the benefits of my eating were clear. My energy was up - nowhere near the deep exhaustion of my first 3 kids, my breast milk was flowing so much better, my moods were even and I had lost most of the bloat in my face.

Visitors commented on how bright my eyes and hair were, and I found that in comparison to my high calorie low nutrition births, I was repairing much faster, needed less sleep, and managed to do so much more than wander around the house like a jersey cow.

If you haven't done it already, week 2 is a good time to test yourself on different meats, unless you don't eat meat.

Like our firewood example, grass fed, organic meat has less "chemical interference" than hormone injected mass produced meat. I do think that it is nearly impossible to find anything that is organic in the true sense of the word, but you can always aim to get the best quality available.

We buy our meat from a butcher at the markets who farms his own cows and chickens, and we buy cryovaced frozen salmon fillets from a wholesaler in Brisbane when we go down there.

While you're at it, have a play with different hard cheeses, I love Danish goats milk fetta in my salads.

Just remember, like the cure for cancer (which is a final road sign in a malnourished life) the cure for a stressed out family is a vegetable based diet.

The only other thing I'll add to this week, is now that your milk is flowing, remember to have a glass of water with you before you start breastfeeding. Once the little munchkin is on the boob, he won't let you stop - and you can go from feeling fine, to feeling like you have the Sahara desert in your mouth with just a few sucks.

I'm still working on this. It's more a note for myself. How can something so simple be so easy to forget!

Week Three

Start Pelvic Floor Exercises

98 out of every 100 mothers that have come through our fitness studio have some degree of pelvic floor degradation.

Amazing, this means that only 2 people in every 100 will regain full control of their PC muscles after birth. We ran a bootcamp for a group of 40 something mums once, and the most amazing thing for us was that while every one of them had a pelvic floor issue, nobody was talking about it. Nobody. As if it were embarrassing to admit.

One day a lady called Kerryn joined up. An ex mounted police officer with a lightning sense of humour. She pronounced in front of all of the other mums. "I hope to hell I don't piss through this nappy, but in case I do, I won't be offended if you give me some room to 'spill'."

Like the sound of horses coming, the murmurs in the crowd of other girls went from quiet to deafening. One mum said she was wearing a nappy too. Another yelled out that she had a tampon and a pad. The lady next to her replied (through tears of laughter) "tampons don't go in the pee hole!"

The funniest thing was how they all tried to make Julius feel awkward.

One of them bent over and flashed her wet bum and said, "that's what happens when you make us skip" to which the rest roared with laugher.

I don't know if Kerryn will ever know of the long term impact of her frank honesty, but I'd like to acknowledge right here that pelvic floor issues are a given. Like stretch marks, you're very likely going to get them - you can manage them well, but don't ever, ever be embarrassed by them.

I mean, seriously, you push a watermelon out of your vagina, and you expect to be able to hold back a little drop of wee?

Week 3 is a great time to start working on rehabilitating your PC muscles. The sooner you get onto them, the better - don't wait until you have a problem, because that may be too late.

I guess the point is that you should *assume* that you are going to have pelvic floor issues, so do something about them now. Don't *hope* that you won't have pelvic floor issues, because doing something about them later can be too late.

The truth is that you should have been working on them from week 1, but after week 2 is where things start to settle down a bit, so I put it here as a last chance reminder. Don't leave it any longer than this.

The surgery that some of our clients have gone through 20 years after having babies (they describe it as 'scaffolding' their vagina) can be quite distressful.

The best exercise for strengthening and tightening the PC muscle for me was what I describe as "picking up" with your vagina. It sounds strange, but it's the only way I could visualise it myself. I imagine that I need to pick something small up with my vagina, like say a grape. I then imagine pulling it up inside me as high as it can go, before reversing the process with control.

To start off with, it felt really uncoordinated, but after a few days of intense concentration, I got it, and it became part of my routine. Once this happened, I did the exercises after I went to the toilet and also in the shower.

I imagined that I needed to save the last drop (sounds gross I know, sorry) but I would imagine using my vagina to pull the last drop of wee back to where it came from.

After I got used to this, I'd try to stop my wee half way through a few times (wow, does this tire out the muscles pretty fast!).

I went to see the pelvic floor specialist physiotherapist that my midwives recommended. I'd suggest doing what you have been taught, after seeing the specialist.

Pelvic floor strengthening is so much more important (timing wise) than any other exercise, and should therefore take priority. Think of it this way, you can always strengthen and tone the rest of your body later. But you can't always do that with your pelvic floor muscles.

Bleeding is lighter

In Week 3, your bleeding should begin to get lighter. For me, this is the signal that my body is finished the birthing process, and is transitioning into the parenting process. Your baby won't be looking like a newborn any more (to you he won't have changed, but compared to when he came out, he should look more like a baby now).

Mobilise

When a baby is born, it is very, very flexible (think about how easily it can put it's foot into it's mouth). For the baby that is because it has very stretchy ligaments.

As time goes by and the baby grows up, the ligaments tighten up to protect and strengthen the joints. From the age of 20, if you don't do something proactive to keep them supple, your connective tissue will tighten up more and more every year to the point that it becomes almost brittle (in old age).

If you don't do something about it, your joints will slowly reduce their range of motion, to the point where as an old woman, you'll feel trapped by your body.

Really old women struggle in the cold, because it takes them so long to get *any* movement from their joints.

For most people, the first they know about the tightening and the reduced range of motion is when they pull a muscle. Once this happens, the process of repairing the muscle while counteracting it with more flexibility in the connective tissue becomes a life long battle.

Giving birth is the equivalent to going back in time (for your ligaments). They are as spongy and supple as a baby. This is because of a hormone called Relaxin. Try it for yourself now - if you couldn't touch your toes before, you're able to do it now with ease!

Use this gift from your baby. I am so mad at myself for sitting around feeling sorry about my body changes after the first 3 kids, I wish that I had used that 'going back in time' to work on my hip and lower back flexibility (or as we call it, mobility).

Just think for a moment about what the possibilities are for you, if you can have dancer like flexibility in your hip joints, in your lower back, in your shoulders.

I'm telling you now that you can! Don't waste another minute; stretch now - your body is saying to you "Do you like this flexibility? Test is out, tell me what you think?"

If you don't do anything about it, your body will just go back to where it was (or worse, your body will go to where most mothers are conditioned to believe it is going).

It is in week 3, because my bleeding stopped, that I consciously began to build the body of my dreams. I've always wanted to be more athletic - I want to run and play with my kids as they get older, I don't want to be the mum who sits on the park bench while her kids play, because she is afraid of hurting herself.

The first step in athleticism is mobility, flexibility. Think of Usain Bolt - if he had restricted movement in any joints of his body, nobody would know his name.

Every single successful athlete on earth works to retain full range of motion in his or her joints. As a mum, you are an Olympic level athlete who never stops and never rests.

It is imperative for you to have full range of motion. If you have been held back by poor flexibility your whole life - use this opportunity now to do something about it!

I did stretches. You can do yoga, pilates, gymnastics, whatever takes your fancy. Do something that will send a message to your body that this flexibility has to become a permanent thing.

And once you start doing stretches, never stop. You probably never will, because your body has this amazing ability to self regulate. It will tell you when you are getting tight and it will nag you to do something about it.

For my hip flexibility, I did a squat hold. Every time I had to change a nappy, I'd put the child on the floor in front of me, and squat right down to do the work. Apart from getting really, really efficient at doing nappies, this was a habit that forced me to keep the post baby flexibility.

For the first few times, I got pins and needles in my legs and felt faint when I stood back up, but now it's just what I do. Other cultures do it to eat or poo, so why can't we?

Just be warned that standing up after a prolonged squat hold can make you feel light headed, so probably not a good idea to do your first few with baby in your arms!

This is a great place to do your pelvic floor hold (or you might fill the nappy yourself!) and I would suggest not doing it on a full bladder.

For my shoulder flexibility, I held a broom handle at each end and passed it over my head and back a few times.

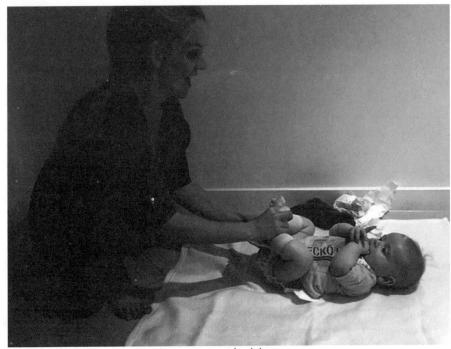

squat hold

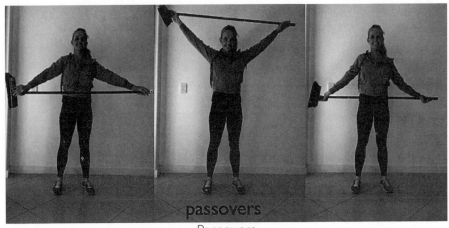

Passovers

While we're on the point of flexibility and injury prevention, now is a good time to start the habit of holding your baby ambidextrously (on each hip equally). I would alternate which side I would feed on, and I also alternate which side I pick them up on.

My osteopath tells me that a lot of women that he treats have issues that stem from only holding a baby on one hip. One side of the body becomes stronger than the other, creating midline instability and pretty bad back injuries down the track.

Exercise in week 3

I still did my walk, which was getting a little longer each time, but in week 3 if you are up to it, start doing some body weight strength exercise.

I aimed to do 10 squats over the toilet every time I had to go. I also did 10 pushups on the edge of the bathroom bench when I brushed my teeth. If I got a chance to, I'd lie underneath the dining room table, and pull myself up (this I could only do about 2 or 3 reps of).

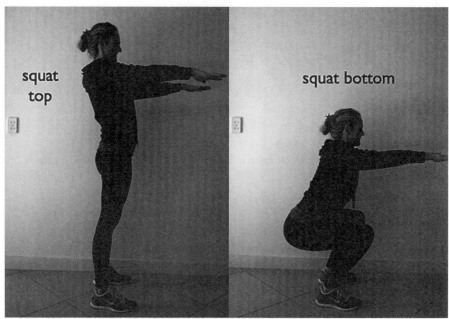

squatting (I spared you the view of the toilet!)

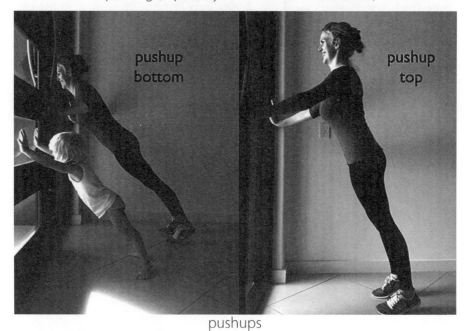

pushups

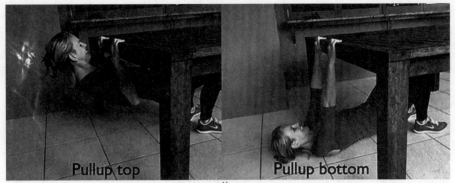

Pullup top | Pullup bottom

pullups

Don't be alarmed at how weak you are in these early stages. The first time I did a squat, I ended up just plopping down - thank goodness I had decided to do it over the toilet, not over the floor!

Remember that you are very flexible for a reason - your strength will come back soon enough; right now just focus on getting a broad range of motion, that is all.

Don't push yourself, you're not going to win the Olympics for decathlon in the 3rd week after having a baby, but what you *can* do is use the time to set yourself up to have the *mobility* of an athletic mum.

Eating in week 3

I still retained the high vegetable diet. I guess at this stage it is important to point out that through my research, I have decided to reduce and eliminate sugar, grains and dairy from my diet altogether. There are plenty of fantastic books that will guide you to your decisions, but our theory on dieting (from our first ever book *Never Diet Again*) is to just try something on yourself - don't take what I do and *expect* that it will work for you. Test it; I'd be happier to hear that you proved it wrong than have people blindly following me without reasons of their own!

My reasons for not having any of these is as follows:

Sugar.

I found that cutting sugar out of my diet altogether changed my moods dramatically. I am reminded of it every time I do sneak some, thinking "this time it will be different"

With sugar, I become an unpredictable monster. I feel like the alcoholic who cannot control his moods on the booze. He knows he's being crazy, but can't stop himself.

As a mum, I refuse to let myself be like that around my kids. It certainly is a work in progress though, because sugar is everywhere, and the shocking thing for me was finding that I have the same reaction with fruit sugar - so I don't eat any fruit on it's own.

If I do have fruit, it will be in my veggie juice (1/2 an apple makes it taste a little sweeter) or in my salad (a few blueberries) once or twice a week.

I did miss fruit to start with, but I don't miss the mood swings and I get all my micronutrients I need from veggies. Now, 15 weeks on and I can't think of the last fruit I did have.

Note: blueberries are the closest fruit to veggies when it comes to their sugar content.

And while I write this, Julius is standing next to me eating a grapefruit. Grapefruits have been a staple for dieters and body builders for years, but I found that the acidity came through in Emmett's nappy and burnt his bum, so I don't eat grapefruit while breastfeeding.

Grains.

The most common grain products are breads and pastas. I find that grains make me tired, lazy and unmotivated. Almost instantly after eating bread, I would feel cloudy in the head. I tried wholemeal and multigrain and found them to be worse (as well as giving me a bonus sore gut). Interestingly, when I ate bread or pasta, Emmett would have a very unsettled sleep.

Dairy.

I only realised after stopping dairy for 7 days that I just felt better without it, so I don't have dairy. Someone asked me the other day how I can make breastmilk without having dairy, and I had to laugh, because I used to think the same thing.

Animals don't drink milk to make milk. Why do we think we have to drink milk to make milk? In fact, why do we have to drink milk at all? The whole calcium theory was thrown out recently as a marketing scam by the dairy industry anyway.

And as Julius likes to say, we are the only animal that still drinks from the teat after we have been weened, and we are drinking it from another animal - kind of disgusting if you think of it that way!

The point here is *not* that dairy, wheat and sugar are bad for you. I found personally that I was better off without them (and you might or might not). The point is that you shouldn't just eat something if the only reason you eat it is *because you always have*. Do your own research and make up your own list of foods that don't agree with you.

Sugar, grains, dairy and soy are great places to start your research journey!

A day of eating for me...

My eating hasn't changed at all since week 3 (I'm now at week 15) and I don't imagine it will change much at all now. I eat pretty much the same thing every day, but I'm not bored with it nor do I crave change.

Now that my micronutrient needs are kept in balance with a rainbow of vegetables, I don't feel that weird about eating the same thing every day any more.

As a mum, it certainly helps me to plan the week ahead, I have gotten good at shopping for what we need, not what we *might feel like*, so wastage is really limited. I also don't live like a Spartan, once or twice a week, I'll go out to lunch with the girls or get takeaway dinner and have something culturally different. Some weeks I will have no meat at all, but generally, it fits into this routine:

Breakfast

A green veggie juice or smoothie with only half an apple and a squeeze of lemon to take the bitterness out of it. The first time I had one of these I had to block my nose, now if it has half an apple in it, it tastes like it has half a cup of sugar in it (such is my sugar sensitivity now!)

A smoothie is blended, a juice is put through the juicer.

OR

2 eggs. (Poached, boiled or scrambled). I make a delicious egg pie in a muffin tray for the kids, just by wrapping a slice of bacon in the base and filling the hole with eggs and garlic chives - the kids love these and they are really easy to make - put in the oven at 250 for about 15 minutes and they are ready.

If I feel like it, I'll have a cup of tea.

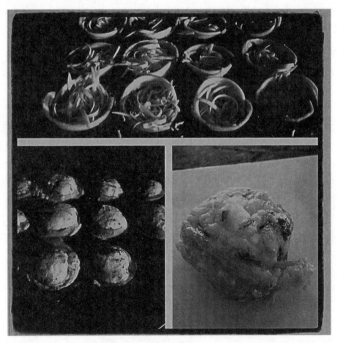

egg pies

Lunch/Dinner

Drinking a veggie juice or smoothie is really, really filling. Because it is jam packed with nutrition, you don't feel hungry for ages. As a result, my lunch and dinner tend to be quite small - not because I want to control my portion size, but because I just feel satiated (like I don't need to eat anything). In fact most days, I feel like I am forcing myself to eat because I have this archaic idea that I need 3 meals a day.

This isn't every day, some days I need more food, and my body tells me by making me hungry - at which point I eat a lot more than normal of my lunch or dinner, which is usually a bowl of steamed veggies or a salad, with steamed salmon or chicken.

Interestingly if I do eat a lot, it is usually the meat that I want, not more veggies. I have never felt hungry eating this way; other than immediately when I sit down to eat.

Snacks

I very seldom have time for snacks, and I feel that if I am making the effort to prepare a snack, I may as well eat a meal. But if I do snack, it's blueberries, almonds or seeds. I have had days where I only eat 3 almonds before feeling full, and days where I have eaten half a packet.

I attest this to my body needing the essential fatty acids in them. Some days it doesn't need any, other days, it must need a lot.

Week Four

Proactive versus Reactive

With my first three kids, the reason I was so disempowered was because I was living a *reactive* life. Waiting for something to happen so that I could *react* to it. For some people, this describes their entire existence.

Someone with a reactive mindset defines their life by what has happened to them. People with victim mentality ("it *always happens to me*" mentality) have a reactive mindset.

A proactive mindset is one where we define our lives by what we do or create *ourselves*.

A proactive mind is a powerful mind. A proactive mind is in control of their lives, a reactive mind is controlled by their lives.

For baby number 4, the biggest part of regaining my power was changing my mindset from reactive to proactive.

And it all starts with time.

Time management

If you don't have a plan for your time, you are at the mercy of someone else's plan for it.

Now when I say time management, I don't mean a colour coded diary and special pens for different categories. These type of time management courses all suck.

I'm going to give you a crash course in effective time management right now, which will have you doing more in one day than you normally would do in a whole week.

Being new mum is the perfect opportunity to become proactive with your life. People expect it of you. Try and implement this stuff at any other time in your life and you are bound to get a few noses bent out of shape.

Time management step 1: Block time thieves

If you steal my money, I can always make it back. If you steal my time, I can never get it back.

Think about the lengths you go to in order to protect your money. Bank accounts, passwords, PIN numbers. If your friend stole money from your purse, you would be very, very upset.

It's a criminal offence to steal other people's money and possessions. You don't go walking around with your purse open, notes flapping in the breeze, do you?

Why on earth then, do we do it with our time?

Think about this. Time, once spent, is gone forever. As your baby grows up, you will begin to look back on photos and wonder how it all went so fast. Already in week 4, the memory of being pregnant is fading.

I'm not talking about wasting time either. That's your prerogative, what I am talking about is allowing other people to steal your time. Once I understood and implemented this concept into my life, I wondered how I had never done it before!

Back to the purse, notes flapping in the wind. You wouldn't do that right? Well, think of all the access points people have that make your time management reactive. For example, your mobile phone. If you carry it around with you, you are inviting someone to call you, and steal your time.

And it's subconscious; it's expected of you. If your phone rings right now, will you stop what you are doing to see who it is, will you answer it?

"It could be important," you say. But it very rarely is. Nobody ever calls you to tell you they have something *for* you. Almost all your calls are from someone who wants something *from* you. Those calls are important, but not to you - they are important to the caller.

If you stop what you are doing and answer the phone, you are saying to yourself, "what I am doing is not as important as what this caller wants. I am not as important to my life as they are".

Time management step 1 then, is to restrict access to yourself in order to block time thieves. Phones are for outgoing calls only. Nobody is going to get offended if you don't answer your phone straight away - that's what message bank is for.

I leave my phone next to my bed all day on silent. I have a home phone that is private and only Julius and Josh know the number to. I know that if it rings, it must be an emergency.

People now know that they will almost always be leaving me a message (which forces them to be concise and get to the point) and that I check my phone at around noon and again at 7pm and will reply to them then, if it is important.

Extrapolate this idea a little. Spend a bit of time thinking about all the access points people have to you. All the ways that you are allowing people to enter your home and steal your time.

Email?

Facebook messenger?

Twitter?

Do you allow people to just 'drop in'?

All of these things put you into a reactive state - they can mess up your routine for your day and put you at the mercy of someone else's plan. If you restrict access to yourself, you control your time. You are proactive.

Time management step 2: Eliminate consumerist behaviour

I used to find myself staring at the computer, half an hour after the kids were meant to wake up, wondering how I got there. I was about a kilometre down the Facebook feed and forgotten what I had come into the office for.

Social media is the ultimate reactive life trap. I am always lost for words when Julius asks me to explain what I actually gain from the time I spend on Facebook scrolling for gossip.

He calls it consumerist behaviour. I call it reactive behaviour. When you just sit in front of the computer, open Facebook and see what comes up. It's like TV. Please don't tell me you have the TV on in the background!

Time management step 3: Do one thing at a time

Once you have eliminated access to yourself and cut out all of your consumerism, you'll be amazed at how much time you actually have! But your mind is a resourceful little devil, it will find things for you to do that will fill in that time AND they won't be fun; they'll be frustrating.

Welcome to the distracted life of a housewife. Laundry half done, hair half done, bottles half washed, emails half typed, book half read…you get the point.

There is a simple solution to this. Just do one thing at a time, at the expense of all else, until it is finished. I was dumbfounded at how fast I could get all the house chores done when I just did them one at a time as opposed to doing them all at once!

Try it, if you have laundry to do and dishes to do and the benches to wipe down, don't try and do them all at once. Just do the dishes until they are done, only then can you start the benches. Once you have cleaned them all, only then can you allow yourself to do the laundry.

I know I'm giving 1950's housewife chores as examples, but let's be realistic, I'm not Angelina and the housework isn't going to complete itself!

There is still one piece to the time management puzzle missing, because for me, even doing these three things, I would waste time. I called it 'planning', but it's probably more accurate to call it indecision...

Time management step 4: Routine

Aah, the holy grail of time management. Routine. If you have all the other steps in place, a routine will take you from reactive, haggard housewife that looks like the witch from Harry Potter, to the powerful, honoured, effective CEO of your own life.

Having a routine eliminates the need for decision. If you know what you are doing for the day, and you do it according to plan, you will have so much more time than you ever had before you had a baby.

Add in the fact that you have more energy because you are eating right and the fact that your hormones reduce your need for sleep and you have the recipe for a proactive, productive life!

2 questions always pop up when we get to this point. The first is "how do I set up a routine" and the second is "what do I do about big projects?"

The answer is simple - instead of making a complicated routine, make a very simple one. One where you block out time to do specific tasks.

Here's mine:

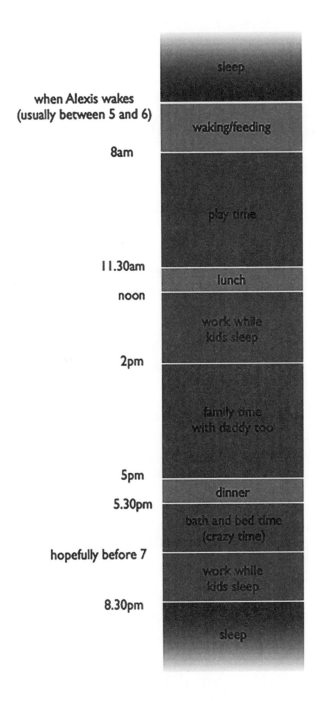

when Alexis wakes
(usually between 5 and 6)

sleep

waking/feeding

8am

play time

11.30am

lunch

noon

work while
kids sleep

2pm

family time
with daddy too

5pm

dinner

5.30pm

bath and bed time
(crazy time)

hopefully before 7

work while
kids sleep

8.30pm

sleep

And this is how it plays out:

5:45 - 6am

Express from 1 breast for 15 mins before I start to feed Emmett.

6am-7am

Breast Feed Emmett on full breast first and then the rest of expressed breast. I use the rest of this hour to get breakfast organised. Sometimes Emmett sleeps until 7, if so, I just feed him then.

7 -7:30am

Breakfast with Alexis, Danté (Emmett in rocker with us)

8am

Brush teeth and dress kids ready for morning to play

8:30 – 9:45

Emmett asleep. Fun play with Alexis and Danté (play doh, colouring in, blocks etc.)

9:30am

Morning Tea for Alexis and Danté

9:45am

Change Emmett and wipe him over with a warm washer, cream him and reswaddle. Alexis and Danté help and love being included.

10am

Feed Emmett. Set Alexis and Danté up in front of wooden puzzles to play in front of me while I feed Emmett.

At 10:45

Express for 15 minutes while Emmett has a lay on the mat and Alexis and Danté play with an activity. (This allows my breast to be empty for exercise).

11am

Give Emmett rest of express breast.

11:20am

Emmett in to cot for his lunchtime sleep.

11:30am

Lunch with Alexis and Danté.

12noon

Alexis and Danté into bed for lunchtime sleep.

12-2:30pm

10 minutes to tidy up from the morning. Do my 15-minute workout, 5 min shower, and work for 2 hours while babies sleep, starting with checking messages and emails. (If I had had a rough nights sleep and was tired, I would work for 1 hour, sleep for 1 hour.)

2:30pm

Feed time/afternoon tea – Wake Alexis and Danté for snack. They snack while I feed Emmett.

3:30pm

Go for my walk with the kiddies. Emmett sleeps and I chat with Alexis and Danté about what they see. If Julius is finished work, he joins us. Great family time.

5pm

Feed Emmett half feed. Alexis and Danté eat dinner. We all sit together and chat while I feed Emmett.

5:45pm

Bath time. Alexis and Danté in Bubble bath. Baby bath set up beside bath so I can bath Emmett at the same time as watching Alexis and Danté.

6pm-6:15pm

Dress Emmett on a padded mat under the warm lights in the bathroom while Alexis and Danté play in the Bath. This way I can watch them.

While Emmett lays dressed on a mat or rocker. I dry and dress Alexis and Danté.

6:15pm

 In a quiet, dim room I feed Emmett the rest of his feed (empty both breasts) while Alexis and Danté lay and drink their sippy cup of rice milk while reading books. A dimmed room helped keep them calm and settled.

6:30pm

Emmett into cot, swaddled.

Brush Alexis and Dante's teeth, get them into their sleeping bags and read them a story together.

6:45pm

Into bed for Alexis and Danté.

6.45 – 7pm

Tidy the house (one thing at a time!)

7 - 7.30pm

Check phone and emails. If time left, check social media.

7:30pm

Work.

8.30pm

Express and then sleep

10pm

Feed Emmett (this feed drops away once he starts on solids)

2am

Feed Emmett (this feed drops away last, when he sleeps through)

Nowadays, I can get more work done in 2 hours than I used to do in a whole week as an employee, but that's a topic for a whole other book.

The point is that for you to be an empowered mum, you have to be a proactive mum. So to recap:

1. Eliminate (or at the very least restrict) access to yourself.
2. Eliminate consumerist behaviour (or at the very least restrict it to a specific block of time)
3. Do one thing at a time until it is complete
4. Create a routine that has blocks of time.

Exercise in Week 4

Now that your bleeding is stopped, and you have managed to get your baby onto the bottle for one of his/her feeds, you can venture out of the house for a run. Run? That's probably a little optimistic - it will be more like a very short plod.

Don't be alarmed at this. You haven't done any real fitness stuff for more than 2 months. That's a long time. But now is a good time to start the habit of exercise. You have blocked a time for it in your routine, so go out and do *something*.

The best time to get fit is when you are really unfit - because the gains in fitness from week to week are massive. One day, you're struggling to walk up the stairs, and a week or two later, your sprinting up them 10 times.

If you stick to your vegetable based diet, and stick to your routine, the weight should be literally falling out of you by now. Until week 4, my weight loss was minimal, but from week 4 to week 8, I got on the scales every morning to a loss.

I've done restrictive diets before and the overwhelming feeling is that you are starving yourself, always hungry, and the weight just fights to stay on you. This time, after 4 weeks of eating a plant based wellness diet, it was as if the fat just gave up and decided to leave.

Week 5 though, is where it all comes together.

Week Five

Week 5 for me was like a reawakening. Clean eating, combined with ruthless time management and strict work on my mobility had me feeling better than I ever had before. I felt euphoric. My sore hips and lower back that I had put up with for the past 5 years literally disappeared overnight.

Compare that to what I felt with all the other births and you would be amazed. By week 5 of each of the other kids, I felt like a dog that has been beaten and beaten and beaten until it just gives up, doesn't even wince when the whip strikes anymore. For 3 births, that is what I felt....

Now though, I felt invincible. I had purpose, I was proactive, I had so much time and I used it well. I was so effective with whatever I did and that is when I started taking notes about what I was doing.

If I could do it, then surely anyone could. I'm nobody special. I mean most people would write me off as a trash, because I had my first baby at 16, I don't have a tertiary education, barely scraped through school and I don't come from money.

But I feel like I've stumbled across a miracle. A miracle that I wish I had found a long time ago, but as Julius says to me; "If you didn't go through hell, you wouldn't have the tools to explain what this turnaround is like."

I'm so grateful for my horrendous, victim, reactive, cowardly behaviour with my first 3 kids; because if it wasn't so bad, I probably wouldn't have bothered to change it.

But the overwhelming point that I want to get across is that if I can do this, and if my friends can do this, then surely you can too - and you know what? You'll probably do a much better job than me!

And the best thing of all?

I no longer have a 'genetically' big butt. I used to train like crazy and crash diet - even with abs; I still had a fat bum. Now, with very little effort, I have the small, shapely bum I have always dreamed off.

When the cool weather of winter finishes, I'm getting into my bikini and walking down the beach with all 4 of my kids and all of my stretch marks. Because I am a mum, I worked hard for them and NOBODY can take that away from me!

Week Six and Beyond

I better not stop at week 5, there are things that you probably need to know about, now that you are the proud queen of your own life. What's it like now? And for all of you whose husbands want to know, when can I have sex again?

I'll cover that in detail soon, but before I do, there are a couple of other milestones that need to be talked about.

Bathing with baby

Once again, this comes from our swimming teacher - in the bath, at around 6 weeks, you should trickle a very small amount of water on your baby's face. When you do, he should get a shocked look on his face, stretch out his arms and basically freeze. This is good. It is the internal reaction (his instinct) to being under water that he needs to have in order to survive.

Doing this every night for his bath will get him used to the feeling, and come time for swimming lessons to start, he won't be afraid of the water - the biggest hurdle to teaching kids how to swim.

It is also a good idea to give them a signal that they get used to. For our kids it is "Emmett… ready…go! And then just a little trickle of water over his face.

Interval training

From week 6, I started to do interval training. Nothing turns a body into a fat burning machine like interval training.

For all three of my other kids, I was told that exercise sours your milk, so I didn't even bother doing it (it was a very convenient excuse) but this time I felt different. My nutrition was good, my body was responding to exercise well, so I gave it a go.

At first I was (once again) shocked at how unfit I was. Our driveway is about 40m long, and moderately inclined. I struggled to run to the top once. But within a couple of weeks of doing it every day, I was doing 10 hill sprints at a time.

Now, Julius and I take the kids to the local lighthouse park most afternoons. He pushes three of them in the chariot while I run next to him. The kids love it, and the older 2 join in for a lot of it, but to me what is so special is that my family can share exercise and vitality as opposed to food.

I always feel so proud of them all as I turn from the top of the hill to see them scattered across the lawn in varying levels of joy!

From week 6 on, I started to swim in the pool. My bleeding stopped well before then, so I could have swum from about week 4, but I just hadn't even thought to swim.

Swimming is a fantastic way to exercise without impact, great news for pelvic floor problems. It is also a great place to do mobility, because without gravity, you can get your body into stretches that would otherwise be impossible to do!

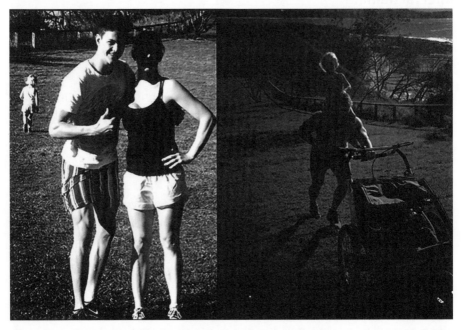

Left: Joshy and me at the bottom (Alexis getting a head start).

Right: Julius with the two little boys in the chariot and Alexis, his jockey

With regards to strength training, I continued to do my squats, pushups and pullups until about week 8, when I felt like I needed more, at which time I just did modified versions of the short (4-15 minute) metabolic conditioning workouts we use in our 8 week athlete program.

Alright, let's talk about sex.

Sex

For the first few babies, the doctors always told Julius and I sternly not to have sex until we saw them again for the 6-week check up. I could swear it is a long running Obstetrics joke, because they always say it with a tip of the head and a wink. We have had 3 different obstetricians, and they all did the same thing.

I imagine them all in their class, like airline hosts practicing the head tip and wink. "No, Darryl, you've got it wrong, tip your head to the left and wink with your *right* eye."

My second piece of evidence for this is that at the 6 week check up, they ask "any pain with intercourse?" as though it is a given that we have ignored their stern warning and gone for it against doctors recommendation.

The third and final piece of evidence is that most people I talk to have resumed sex before 6 weeks. I know one lady who fell pregnant two weeks post partum!

So, according to my investigative research, I believe that the 6-week warning is there to help make it easier. It can be awkward and sore, and because of the prolactin from breastfeeding, the vagina can be quite dry. If you and your husband know that you are not meant to have sex for 6 weeks, and when you simply cannot wait any longer, you will be more careful, and should it hurt too much, you won't feel bad about pulling out and waiting a few more days.

But here's the good news. Because of all the new blood vessels you have downstairs, sex after birth for most women is much better than before. Even our bootcamp girls all mostly agreed (except the two ladies who had a C section) that their sex lives were so much better after childbirth.

While you'll have much less opportunity to make love (you certainly won't have time for long drawn out love making sessions for some time), the sex you do have will be more rewarding and more delicious.

Most women say that they are able to have multiple orgasms after birth, where before this was a struggle. Bonus!

When to have sex for the first time after birth is up to you, but most people suggest that you wait until you've stopped bleeding, or at least until the bleeding goes from red to pink.

Use plenty of lubricant, and take it slow. The potential for pain is when the penis enters you for the first time, or when it is in deep. So take it slow.

I find the best positions to be in are where I control the depth and the angle. Riding on top is best, and gives a great view of your now much bigger breasts for your husband.

Just be warned that if your husband stimulates your breasts, your milk will come down and they will spray everywhere. This can be quite exciting and adds another kinky element to your lovemaking, but it is also messy.

Some couples do find it hard to include your breasts in sex, because of this feeling that they are the baby's feeding station now, and fondling, kissing and sucking them are just weird. If this is the case, plan on having a shower after sex, or at the least cleaning your boobs with a warm washer to separate sex from feeding.

After the first few times, you can incorporate your pelvic floor exercises into your lovemaking. This is where you can step them up a notch, and your husband can really benefit. After you are warmed up and well lubricated, slow right down and consciously try to squeeze him with your vagina wall, imagine trying to hold his penis, and prevent it from moving. You both will really, really enjoy this exercise. It's the gateway to multiple orgasms for you, and the look on your husbands face will be priceless when he feels your new skill for the first time.

An old married couple once told me that to keep your marriage strong through children, you have to always remember that when your kids one day leave, it will be just the two of you again. So work on your relationship. Work on your sex life.

Go out on date nights with your husband. Organise a babysitter and go out to a local hotel for one night – you feel like you're on holiday, but you're 10 minutes from home if you're needed. Just keep in the back of your mind, this baby will one day grow up and leave. If you work on your relationship with your husband now, he will still be there through it all.

Julius and I always talk about the married couple who marry for love, have kids and through time and neglect, the only thing they have left in common is the kids they share. I certainly don't want to have the kids grow up and leave, only to look across the table to a complete stranger, who once was my best friend, lover and husband.

You are the Queen

I hope that you have enjoyed this book, and I hope that you feel empowered and strong, like a mother should be. I really have kept it short and to the point because I didn't want to steal any of your time by 'fattening out' the book. I wanted every minute you spent reading to be an investment of your time, rather than time wasted.

One final message I'd like to get in here before wrapping up and taking any more of your precious time is that you are perfect for you. Nobody knows your body like you do, not me, not your mother, not a doctor. You.

You are the expert when it comes to you, and as Dr Seuss says:

"Today you are You, that is truer than true.
There is no one alive who is Youer than You."

Refuse to be the slave in your life; you are the queen who understands that to look after yourself first means that you are better equipped to look after everyone else.

Go out and be inspirational, be proud of your mummy badges, be proud of your baby, be proud of your marriage, be proud of what you have achieved so far. You are powerful, you are sexy, you are the queen.

You are a mum!

A few recipes

Egg Pies (Makes 12 egg pies)

Ingredients:

- 12 pieces of rindless bacon
- 12 eggs
- Handful of Fresh garlic chives finely sliced
- Inch slice white goats milk cheese (crumbled)
- Diced fresh tomato

Method

Preheat oven on 200C.

Slice bacon long ways in half and line the outside of each muffin cup with bacon halves.

Add eggs and all other ingredients to mixing bowl and beat with fork. Pour into each muffin cup. Feel free to add other ingredients like mushrooms etc.

Put muffin tray in oven for 15 minutes.

Allow 10mins to cool.

Can be eaten warm or cold as a snack and kids LOVE them

Green Veggie Juice or Smoothie

Ingredients:

- 1 cucumber
- 2 zucchini
- 4 broccoli florets
- 3 celery sticks
- 6 kale stalks de-stemmed
- Half a green apple
- Squeeze a quarter fresh lemons

Method:

FOR JUICE – add all above ingredients to juicer. We have a Juicepresso slow press juicer. A slow press juicer is best.

FOR SMOOTHIE - add all ingredients to blender. This creates a thicker consistency and I find I am fuller for longer.

Rainbow of blanched veggies

Ingredients:

(choose a rainbow of veggies you love, but this is what I have and my kids love it too)

- 6 florets of broccoli
- 6 florets of cauliflower
- 6 halved beans
- 6 button mushrooms
- 1 sliced carrots
- 1 sliced zucchini
- 3 brussels sprouts
- 1 squash cut in quarters
- corn, cut into 3 pieces
- Pinch of Himalayan sea salt (optional)

Method:

Bring saucepan of water to boil.

Add all above ingredients for 3mins.

Drain into colander and put into bowl with a pinch of Himalayan sea salt if desired.

My favourite Green Salad

Ingredients:

(the key to this salad being delicious is to cut everything fine – big chunks will make you gag)

Kale de-stemmed and finely chopped.

2 cups of baby spinach leaves. finely chopped.

1 quarter of a red, green and yellow capsicum. Finely chopped.

Tablespoon of activated sunflower and pepita seeds.

1 quarter of a finely chopped apple or a whole kiwi fruit.

½ beetroot grated

1 carrot grated

1 cup of finely chopped cabbage.

Method:

Mix... lol

Activated nuts and seeds

When you water a seed, it takes about 3 days to sprout a little stem or root. In those three days, the seed still looks like a seed, but inside, it is turning into a plant. One day, it is a seed, a couple of days later, it is a plant.

When it is a seed, it is in a state of protection against digestion. Remember that most seeds are meant to pass through the digestive system unchanged. this is how most seeds or nuts are eaten by humans.

When it is a plant, it is in a state of growth. It is using up all the resources around it to grow. Birds love these.

In between seed and plant is a state called "activated". The seed is shedding it's protective layer, and using all the stored energy inside itself to change into a plant. Eating activated seeds will give all that potential energy and goodness to *you*.

So here's how to do it:

Soak some nuts or seeds overnight in water (some people like to add a tblspoon of Himalayan sea salt).

Drain, and then spread out on a baking tray or tray of dehydrator.

Dry in oven or dehydrator for 12 – 24 hours. (Dehydrate at lowest temperature possible on your oven)

Eat them within the day. If you don't eat them within 2 days, you will be eating a dead seed.

Note: We use our dehydrator but oven is fine if you don't have a dehydrator, we tried laying them out on trays in the sun, but the birds ate them

Talk to us!

We'd love to hear from you, please let us know if and how this book has helped you. Just shoot us a quick email at

sharnyandjulius@sharnyandjulius.com

Thankyou for taking the time to read our book!

Sharny and Julius Kieser

You can also follow us on social media by searching:

sharnyandjulius

The Kiesers